LOUISE ...DES

Hip to Pain?

Simple Guide to Prepare For and Recover From Total Hip Replacement Surgery

Copyright © 2022 by Louise Endes

All rights reserved. No part of this publication may be reproduced, stored or transmitted in any form or by any means, electronic, mechanical, photocopying, recording, scanning, or otherwise without written permission from the publisher. It is illegal to copy this book, post it to a website, or distribute it by any other means without permission.

Louise Endes asserts the moral right to be identified as the author of this work.

Louise Endes has no responsibility for the persistence or accuracy of URLs for external or third-party Internet Websites referred to in this publication and does not guarantee that any content on such Websites is, or will remain, accurate or appropriate.

Designations used by companies to distinguish their products are often claimed as trademarks. All brand names and product names used in this book and on its cover are trade names, service marks, trademarks and registered trademarks of their respective owners. The publishers and the book are not associated with any product or vendor mentioned in this book. None of the companies referenced within the book have endorsed the book.

First edition

This book was professionally typeset on Reedsy.
Find out more at reedsy.com

Contents

1	INTRODUCTION	1
2	HOW TO KNOW SURGERY IS RIGHT FOR YOU	3
	Living With Pain and Limited Mobility	3
	Impacting Your Quality of Life	5
	Choosing Your Surgeon	7
3	BEFORE SURGERY: THINGS TO DO	9
	Dental & Medical Clearances	9
	Prepare Your Mind & Body	10
	Prepare Your Home	12
	Prepare Your Family	15
	Find An Escort	16
	Legal Check-Up	17
4	SURGERY DAY: WHAT TO EXPECT	19
	Anterior vs Posterior Approach	19
	Same Day Physical Therapy	23
	Inpatient vs Outpatient	24
5	AFTER SURGERY: TIPS & TIMELINE	26
	Weeks One to Three - Patience and Pain Management	26
	Weeks Four to Six - Persistence and Progress	30
	Weeks Seven to Twelve - Perseverance and Purpose	32
6	CONCLUSION	33
	Celebrate Success!	33
7	RESOURCES	35

1

INTRODUCTION

The first sign happened when I got up from my desk. I couldn't stand up. My hip felt as if it was locked up. I had to sit back down and slowly stand to be able to straighten it out. Then this would happen in mid stride. Walking through the grocery store parking lot, I stopped suddenly because my hip would lock up.

Like most people, I brushed it off as getting older. Fast forward a couple years and it was happening more frequently accompanied by pain.

Throbbing, burning pain that lasted.

Pain that would wake me up at night.

Pain that started limiting my everyday activities including things that made me happy, like hiking with my husband and dogs. Exercising at home has always been a big part of my life and that was limited too.

The physical turmoil began affecting me mentally. It was no longer just the quality of my function but the quality of life overall that was impacted.

When this first began, I did see my doctor and was sent to Physical Therapy. Two years later, when I went back, they took an x-ray. The deterioration in the joint showed the head of my thigh bone (the femur) rubbing against the pelvic socket,

The doc did not hesitate: "If you wanted to proceed with total hip replacement, I would schedule you without hesitation."

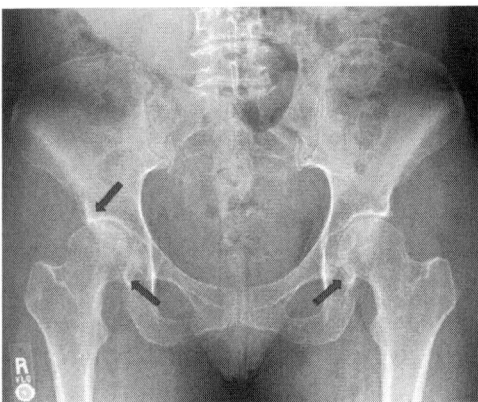

Note: I had my right hip replaced. However, my left hip is showing signs of degeneration also.

DISCLAIMER: Information provided is for educational purposes, based upon my personal experiences not as an expert. Please consult a medical professional for advice, diagnosis and treatment specific to your circumstances.

2

HOW TO KNOW SURGERY IS RIGHT FOR YOU

Living With Pain and Limited Mobility

Questions you might be asking yourself:

- Why am I experiencing pain with certain movements?
- Where is the pain actually coming from?
- What can I do, besides surgery, to alleviate the pain?

Of course, you want to ask your doctor these questions too. Likely, it's arthritis affecting your joints.

What is hip arthritis? In layman's terms, it is joint inflammation. Arthritis is a combination of "arthro" a greek term for joint and "itis" a suffix meaning inflammation.

Side Note: Whenever you see 'itis' it is swelling or inflammation of that area. For example tendonitis is tendon inflammation. Gastritis is inflammation of the stomach lining.

According to John Hopkins, "Hip arthritis is deterioration of the cartilage of the hip joint. The hip is a ball-and-socket joint with the ball at the top of the thighbone (the femoral head). The ball is separated from the socket (the acetabulum) by cartilage. The cartilage acts as a slippery coating between the ball and the socket that allows the ball to glide and rotate smoothly when the leg moves. The labrum, a strong cartilage that lines the outer rim of the socket, provides stability.

When cartilage in the hip is damaged, it becomes rough. Thinning of cartilage narrows the space between the bones. In advanced cases, bone rubs on bone, and any movement can cause pain and stiffness. When there is friction at any point between bones, it can also lead to bone spurs — bone growths on the edges of a bone that change its shape."

Personally, I never thought of my hip pain and limited mobility as 'arthritis'. When my knuckles hurt on my hand, I considered that arthritis (because that's what my mom would also say jokingly… "Arthur's back.") Well, it's a similar occurrence just on a much bigger scale involving a joint that bears the weight of our body.

Your hip joint is one of the largest, strongest, weight-bearing joints in your body. And, like the shoulder, it is a ball-and-socket joint which allows it to move in all directions.

Not all arthritis is created equal:

Osteoarthritis (osteo=bone + arthr=joint + itis=inflammation) is one of the main types of joint pain. It is the wear-and-tear of the cartilage in the joint that keeps the femur head (ball) articulating (moving) normally in the hip socket. When the cartilage breaks down, it becomes thinner or non-existent and fails to provide the cushion that the joint needs between the ball and the socket. That is when you begin feeling pain and limited mobility - the head of the femur is literally scraping against the bone around the socket.

Osteoarthritis is a degenerative condition. Therefore, if it is left untreated, it will create further dysfunction and serious disability over time.

Rheumatoid Arthritis may feel similar but has a different cause. Rheumatoid Arthritis (RA) is when the body's immune system attacks the connective tissue that makes up the membrane lining your joints. RA isn't specific to the hip joint. This may be the cause of pain and stiffness in one or more joints.

Rheumatoid Arthritis is an autoimmune condition that is chronic. Total hip replacement may be necessary, especially if you've been dealing with this pain long-term. However, joint replacement will not address the underlying cause, therefore, additional treatments are suggested. Such as lifestyle changes, therapy, and medication.

Impacting Your Quality of Life

The human body is beyond amazing at adapting to all kinds of circumstances. It's built to survive, even when we intentionally abuse it.

Homeostasis is our body's thermostat that regulates our bodily functions. That's the physical aspect, but what about the mental and emotional toil?

The brain is an organ. And, like the rest of the body, it will <u>try</u> to keep you mentally strong.

Over time though, no matter how well your mind is coping, your quality of life will inherently deteriorate. In my opinion, this is a critical sign that surgery is a must.

Quality of life: **the degree to which an individual is healthy, comfortable, and able to participate in or enjoy life events. ~Britannica**

To measure the degree of your quality of life, ask yourself:

- Am I able to do activities that make me happy (hike, walk, sit in a movie theater)?
- Does the limited mobility affect my performance of everyday tasks (home, work, social)?
- Has chronic pain affected my attitude? my relationships? my goals? my outlook on life?
- Do I feel like nothing I try is giving me any relief?

I knew once I honestly answered these questions – it was time to schedule my total hip replacement surgery.

Choosing Your Surgeon

Once you decide to move forward with having surgery, it is exciting *and* scary at the same time.

"Hippies" (people who've had a total hip replacement) will rave and tell you how happy you're going to be that you did it. It's a life changer. Yay! (insert squeals of excitement because you feel hope again)

But then you Google 'total hip replacement'. Ack! They're going to do what with my what? Day surgery? and just like that, excitement is replaced with fear.

TRUST the process.

- Over 450,000 total hip replacements are performed every year in the United States.
- It's reported that hip replacement is one of the most successful operations.
- The anterior approach, that many surgeons perform now, allows you to get up and walk the same day as the surgery.

Now to find an orthopedic surgeon you can also trust. Ask them:

- How many hip replacements surgeries have you performed?
- Is this procedure something they specialize in?
- Do you do the anterior or posterior approach? (more on this later)
- What material will be used?
- Do they have patient reviews that you can look at?

Here is a site that provides valuable information to get you started on your search for doctors in your area: https://www.md.com

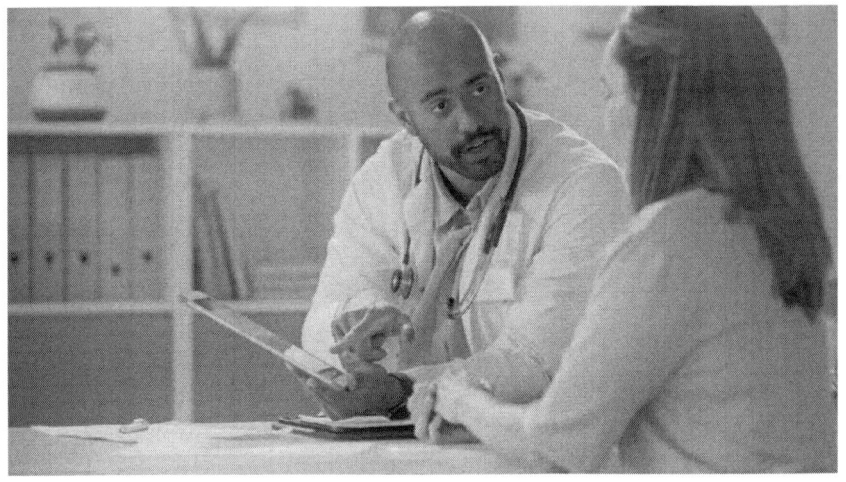

3

BEFORE SURGERY: THINGS TO DO

You've chosen your surgeon. Great! Did you know that most doctors require a couple clearances <u>before</u> they will actually <u>schedule your surgery</u>.

If you're like me, once you decide to do something you just want to get it done. I wanted to get the journey to recovery and an activity-filled, pain-free life started immediately.

That's not how it works.

Preparation really begins months before your surgery.

Dental & Medical Clearances

As mentioned before, hip replacement surgery itself is a highly successful operation. The biggest area of concern is post-operative infection

If dental procedures are required, it is highly recommended (and often required) to have them completed prior to surgery – including a cleaning. Bacteria from dental work can enter the bloodstream. This bacteria will seek out vulnerable areas in the body which include the hip joint prosthesis (your new hip hardware.)

Most likely you will be asked to get a dental clearance form signed by your dentist.

Along those same lines, certain medical clearances will need to be obtained. Depending on your medical history, you may require some or all of the following:

- Blood work: complete blood count (CBC) and comprehensive metabolic panel (CMP)
- Blood work: hemoglobin A1C - if diabetic
- Electrocardiogram - if history of or potential for heart disease
- Cervical X-Rays - if history of or potential for rheumatoid arthritis
- Physical exam - BMI 40 or less
- List of medications
- No steroid injections in the hip within 3-6 months of surgery

Prepare Your Mind & Body

Just like choosing the right doctor for your operation, you also need the right mindset and a body that is ready to work with you, not against you once the recovery phase begins.

Mind:

- **Check your calendar** and be aware of any responsibilities that need to be taken care of leading up to your surgery date and anything that might come after surgery. Removing these distractions and/or stressors will allow you to give yourself grace and time to recover properly.
- **Connect with others** that have had a total hip replacement. Hearing their experiences will help alleviate any anxiety that might be creeping in.
- **Reiterate – to your brain –** that this is going to be a process, not an event. It helps to prepare mentally by letting your mind's eye, your brain, envision that process. Your mind can be either an ally or an enemy.

Body:

- **Losing weight** may be needed or desired. The hip is a weight-bearing joint, so being a healthy weight will assist the progress you make in your recovery.
- **Eating nutrient-dense foods** will also help reduce inflammation and aid recovery. If you don't already eat relatively healthy, dig into this topic to educate yourself on what is going to help your body help you.
- **Fiber deserves its own bullet point.** Most people do not eat enough fiber anyway. The medications you are going to received during and after the surgery WILL constipate you. You want to get ahead of this so start supplementing your diet with good, quality fiber.
- **Quit smoking.** Some doctors require you to be tobacco-free for 6 weeks prior to your surgery.

- **Physical therapy** before hip replacement is a great idea. Your recovery, and overall well-being, will benefit immensely from strengthened muscles, improved flexibility and the confidence boost that comes with it.

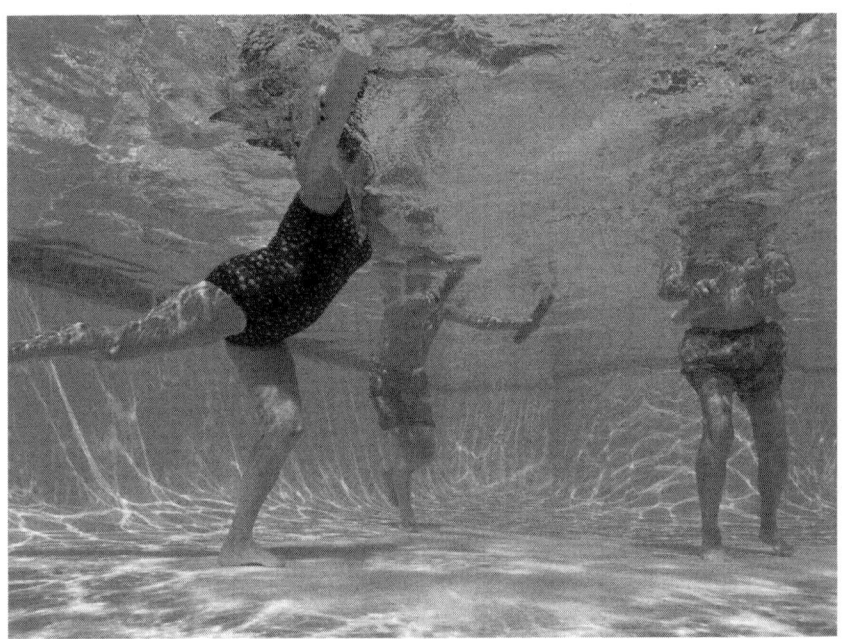

Prepare Your Home

This may or may not apply to you, but first things first:

- have a stable environment to go home to. Are there family or roommate issues that need to be resolved, or unsafe conditions that need to be eliminated. You will have a hard time healing in an environment that is not safe or healthy itself.

You may have a caregiver or family that will take care of preparing meals.

- If not, stock your cupboards and fridge with easy to make foods you enjoy. Continue eating healthy options which will provide your body with the nutrients it needs for the healing process.
- Got animals? Be sure to stock up for them too.

Home medical equipment to have in place are:

- Raised toilet seat
- Bath/shower chair
- Grab bar for shower/bath
- Walking aids (these are not always provided by the hospital) i.e. walker, crutches, cane
- Lightweight reacher
- Hospital bed, if necessary*

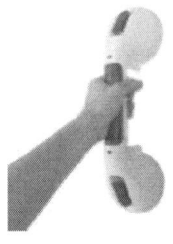 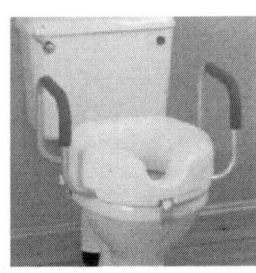 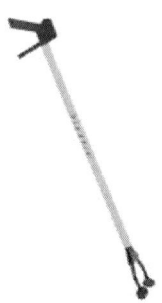

*With the anterior approach hip replacement, you will be able to walk up and down stairs from Day 1. I *could* make it to my upstairs bedroom, but I was not going to sleep in a bed with dogs, so a hospital bed in the living room was essential for me. They are very affordable to rent.

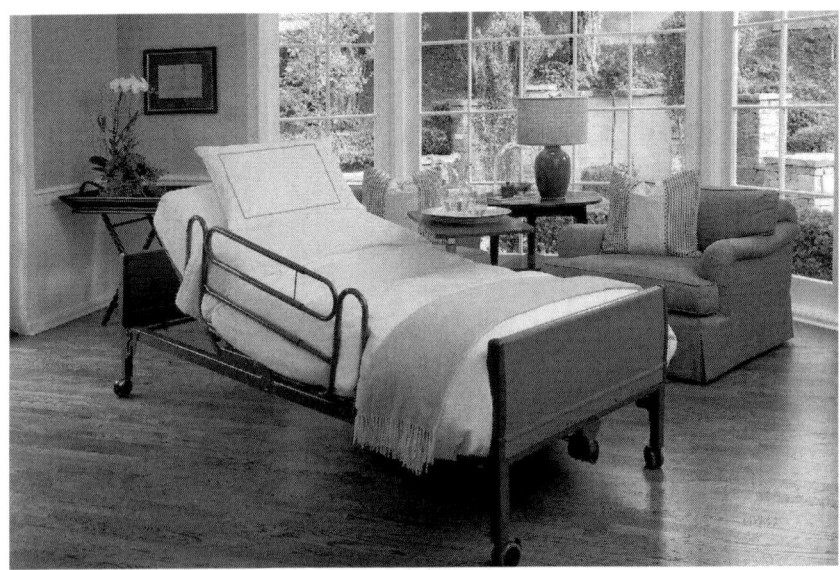

Additional considerations that make your first few weeks easier:

- loose fitting items of clothing to wear
- stable, slip on footwear
- bath wash shower wipes
- books to read
- TV shows recorded to watch
- download a meditation app (great for healing)
- a craft project or puzzle ready to start or finish.

Prepare Your Family

If your family is used to you doing a lot of the everyday things around the house, like cooking, laundry, grocery shopping, dropping kiddos off at school, taking care of pets, etc., involve them in all of the suggestions above.

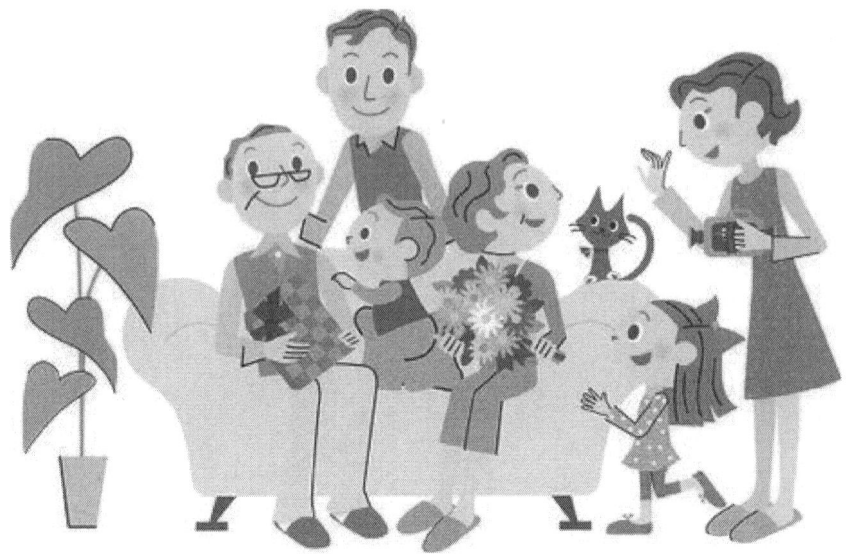

Get your family mentally and physically ready to go through the recovery process with you.

Find An Escort

No, not that kind of escort. You will need a reliable friend or family member that will bring you home after surgery and will stay with you for the first 1-2 days. In my experience, it took about 24-48 hours to figure out how to move around safely and do things for myself.

This may also be the same person who will give your rides to and from your physical therapy appointments.

Legal Check-Up

Another disclaimer: I am not a legal expert. I recommend you speak with a lawyer and/or financial advisor regarding the suggestions below.

As adults, these are things we really should have in order anyway, but for most of us, it doesn't happen until we are faced with our mortality:

Living Will:

- Designate who will have medical power-of-attorney in the event you are not able to make medical decisions for yourself. This type of document allows you to express your wishes ahead of time.
- We pray we never need this, but having one in place will provide peace of mind for you, and in the event it needs to be executed, it will relieve the burden on the person(s) you designate.

Last Will and Testament:

- Life is brief and fragile and loaned to us for a short while. We must always think about what and who we leave behind. It is not our loved ones' duty to determine what to do with our personal belongings, or to determine who gets what. That is your job to do before it is needed.
- It can be as simple as creating a will from a site like www.legalzoom.com

Life Insurance:

- Life insurance is not for you or about you. It is for those we leave behind. If your family depends on your income, they won't ever be able to replace you, but a life insurance policy will help to replace your income.
- Final arrangements cost on average $10,000. Yeah, you may be saying "I'm just going to be cremated and have my ashes spread in the mountains." That is great. In fact, that was my mom's wish. As the kids left behind, we honored that but we also wanted a headstone to place beside our father's. That cost could have been covered by a final expense life policy. Instead we had to pull from our savings to cover that cost.

Sorry I had to go there, but this chapter is about being fully prepared.

Keep reading, you're just getting to the juicy stuff!

4

SURGERY DAY: WHAT TO EXPECT

Your home is ready. Your family is ready. Your affairs are in order. YOU are ready!

Anterior vs Posterior Approach

I touched on this earlier. Anatomically, anterior is the front of your body and posterior is the back of your body. Below is information on the differences, so that you can make an informed decision with your doctor on which is right for you.

Up until the 1970s, hip replacements were always done using a posterior approach. There are advantages and disadvantages for both methods.

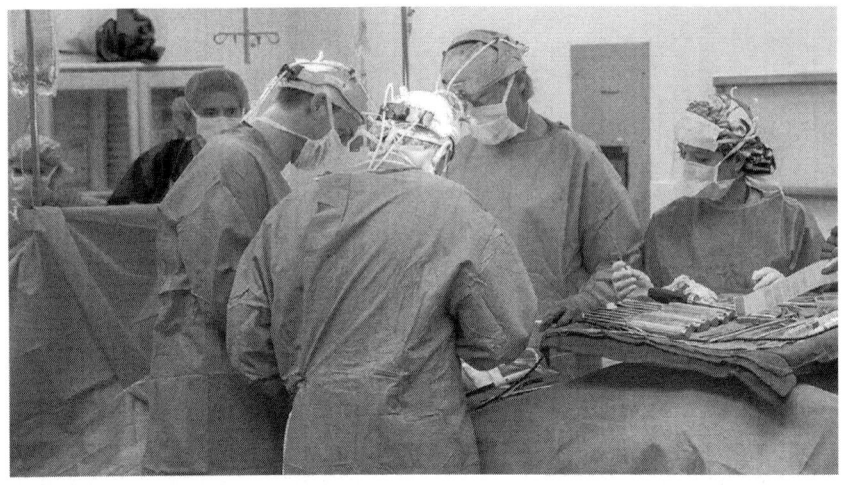

Anterior Advantages:

Typically, when making the incision, which is actually on the side of your hip, the surgeon will be able to access the hip from the front aspect without cutting any muscles.

- Less damage to muscles
- Less postoperative pain
- Faster recovery
- Fewer post surgical precautions

Anterior Disadvantages:

You had me at less pain and faster recovery. But it's important to also know the potential downsides.

- A greater chance of issues with incision healing
- Typically not suitable for obese or very muscular people
- It is a technically demanding surgery.

In making my personal decision, the pros outweigh the cons.

- I could take steps to help reduce the possibility of an infection of my incision.
- I am not obese or very muscular
- I chose a surgeon with proven experience with anterior hip replacement

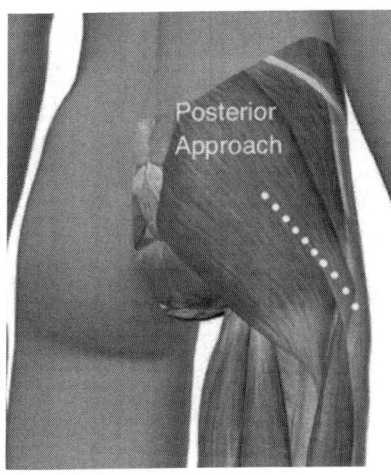 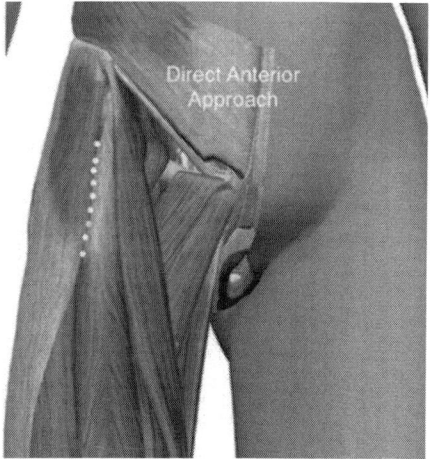

Posterior Advantages:

Because the incision is made on the back side of the hip, it provides the doctor with a better view of and easier access to the hip joint.

Posterior Disadvantages:

The advantage above becomes a disadvantage when considering the muscles and soft tissue affected with this approach, including:

- Tensor fascia lata - a large tendon that attaches at the top of the hip connects with the iliotibial band that runs down along the side of the thigh to help stabilize the knee
- Large gluteal muscle which helps stabilize the pelvis as we stand and move
- Deeper, smaller rotator muscles which assist the gluteus muscles in rotational movements

Additionally:

- Recovery takes longer
- More restrictions on movement in early recovery
- Greater chance of dislocation
- More pain as the cut muscles and soft tissue heal

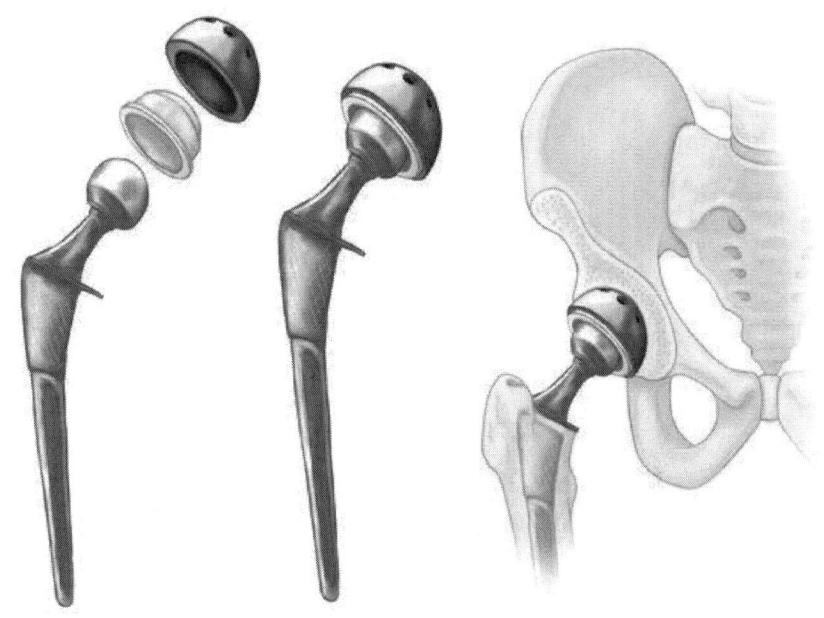

Same Day Physical Therapy

Like most people, when they told me I would be up and walking around the same day of the surgery I was astonished. In fact, anterior hip replacement surgeries are considered day surgery. You could go to the hospital in the morning, have total hip replacement surgery, and go home that night.

Some joint surgeries require complete immobilization as the affected area heals and becomes more stable. Not with the hip.

A physical therapist will visit you in your hospital room once the anesthesia wears off and will have you up, out of bed, trying out your new hip. The first rule of recovery is to keep yourself mobile.

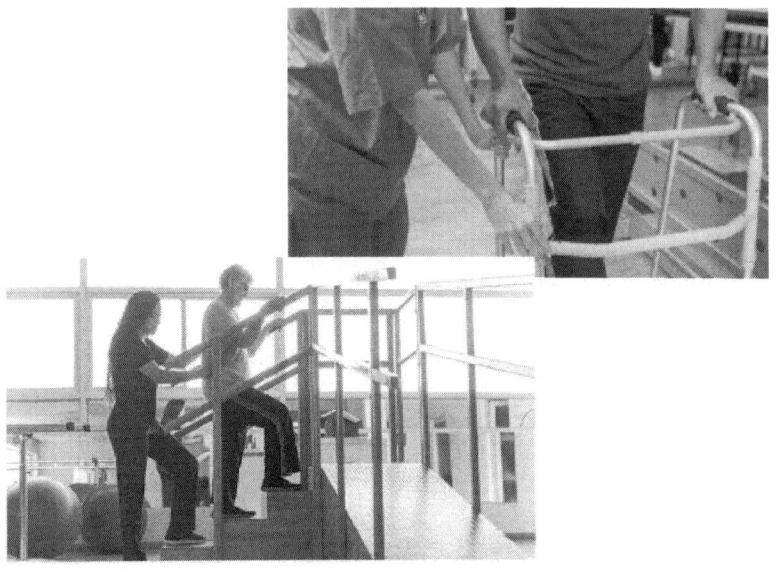

Inpatient vs Outpatient

I mentioned that this can be a day surgery, also called outpatient surgery. The hospital physical therapist will have you:

- walking with a walker up and down the hospital hallways,
- going up and down stairs using a handrail and also using a single crutch, and
- they'll ask you questions to ensure you're set up for a safe and successful recovery at home.

Then you're ready to be discharged. Amazing, right?

SURGERY DAY: WHAT TO EXPECT

Some reason you might be admitted to the hospital for at least an overnight stay:

- If you're not able to do physical therapy (PT) that same day as surgery. In my case, the anesthesia made me very dizzy when I stood upright so my PT was postponed to the next morning.
- If your postoperative blood work presents potential issues. The hospital will want to monitor you until your blood panel readings are within normal ranges.
- If your incision appears infected.
- If you are showing signs of a blood clot.

5

AFTER SURGERY: TIPS & TIMELINE

Weeks One to Three - Patience and Pain Management

You're home, now what? Take it easy, but keep it moving.

In the first few weeks, your primary focus will be staying mobile while managing your pain. It can be easy physically and mentally to just be a couch potato, but that immediate reward will actually hamper and potentially extend the healing process.

Physical Therapy: Prior to going home from the hospital, it's a good idea to already have your physical therapy appointments scheduled for the first 30 days.

You will also need someone to drive you to and from your appointments. Depending on which hip you had replaced, the amount of time before you can drive varies:

If your left hip was replaced (and you don't drive a stick shift), you can resume driving as soon as you've stopped taking narcotic pain medication.

If your right hip was replaced, it will be 3-6 weeks depending on your recovery progress. You must be able to react quickly which will require quick movement of your hip and leg. You want to be able to do this for your and others safety plus you do not want to set back your recovery by straining the joint and soft tissue.

Pain Management: Before you leave the hospital you will be prescribed a few different medications. It's important to stay ahead of your pain. If you try to 'handle' the pain with no meds, and it gets too intense, getting on top of the pain and getting relief will be harder.

I'm all for natural healing and addressing the cause of pain and symptoms instead of just medicating it. However, after surgery, I'm a big proponent of reducing the stress and inflammation using medication, so that your body can direct its energy to the healing process.

<u>Narcotic pain medication</u> - the only thing I will say about this is…it's a narcotic. Everyone will be different with their pain tolerance and recovery, but set your intention to stop taking narcotic meds as soon as you are able. There are other ways to alleviate the pain, which are outlined below.

Important note: if you are having trouble managing your pain, let your doctor know. If you have any addictive tendencies, let your doctor know and find alternatives besides narcotics.

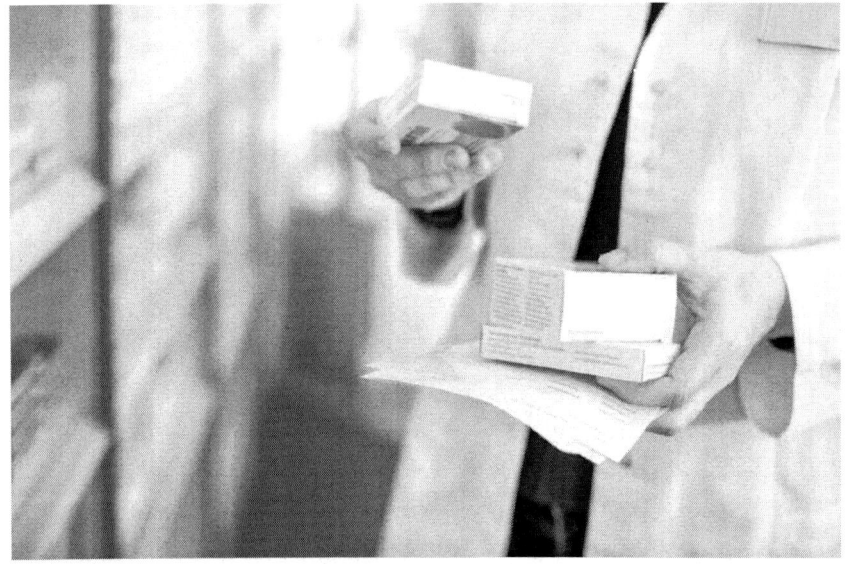

Ibuprofen or acetaminophen - can be used in conjunction with the narcotic pain reliever.

Aspirin - is prescribed for the first 6 weeks, usually until your second post-op appointment with the surgeon. Unless you're on blood thinners already, aspirin will reduce the possibility of blood clots forming.

Rest - you do want to keep the new joint mobile, but rest is required to manage the pain. This is a good time to use ice.

Ice - is one of the best ways to manage pain and aids the healing process. Oftentimes, you will be given a device which looks like a small cooler with a hose coming out of it. You attach the hose to a pad that you place around the hip area. The device is filled with water and ice. It circulates the ice cold water through the pad reducing inflammation which will reduce the pain.

Elevation - a basic element of pain management. When you're resting and icing, prop your lower leg on a few pillows. Elevation will help reduce swelling of the lower leg and knee area and will increase blood circulation toward the hip that aids natural healing.

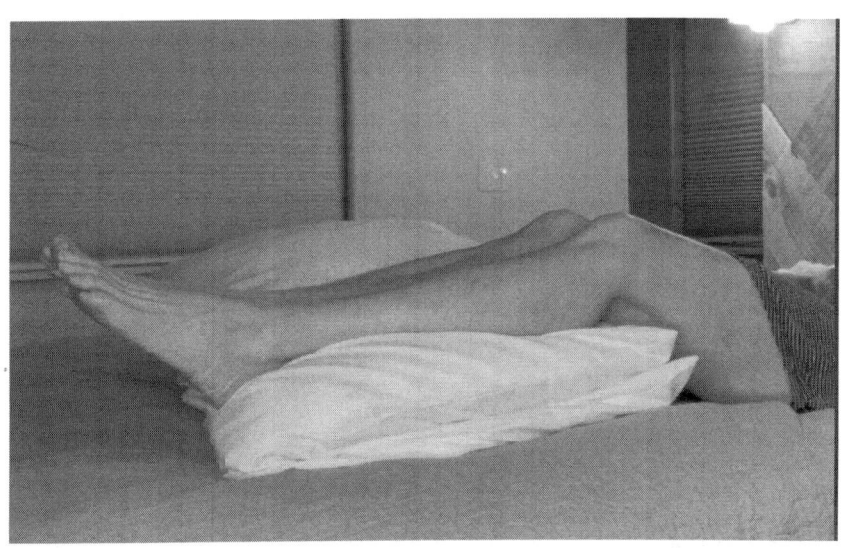

Patience: *"Patience is not the ability to wait, but the ability to keep a good attitude while waiting." ~unknown*

If you've ever healed from an injury before, you might experience what I did. About two weeks in, I:

- had chucked the walker and the crutch.
- was getting around pretty good with a cane
- was feeling stable on stairs
- had my pain under control
- was making great progress each day, thanks to physical therapy,
- **was going stir-crazy!!**

I wanted to be fully-functional, getting on with all the things I dreamed of doing once my hip was replaced.

Stay patient. Continue to trust the process. You will be amazed at how much progress you make each day moving forward. Without patience, you may try to do too much too soon. Nobody has the time or patience for a setback.

Weeks Four to Six - Persistence and Progress

For most people, this is where the magic of medicine really starts taking on life.

Remember the suggestions in Things To Do Before Surgery, specifically preparing your mind and body? That effort, along with postoperative PT, is really paying off now in Weeks 4-6.

You should be able to walk without a cane, and you can begin enjoying everyday activities, virtually pain free. If you are still experiencing some pain at this point, do not let it get you down. It just means you probably have a little more healing today.

AFTER SURGERY: TIPS & TIMELINE

Stay patient but persistent.

Persistence: "Change is hardest at the beginning, messiest in the middle and best the end." ~Robert Sharma

---

You're in the middle.

Don't settle for feeling better.

You took a giant (painful) leap of faith when you decided to have this surgery.

Of course, we want to feel better but this is your opportunity to feel your best!

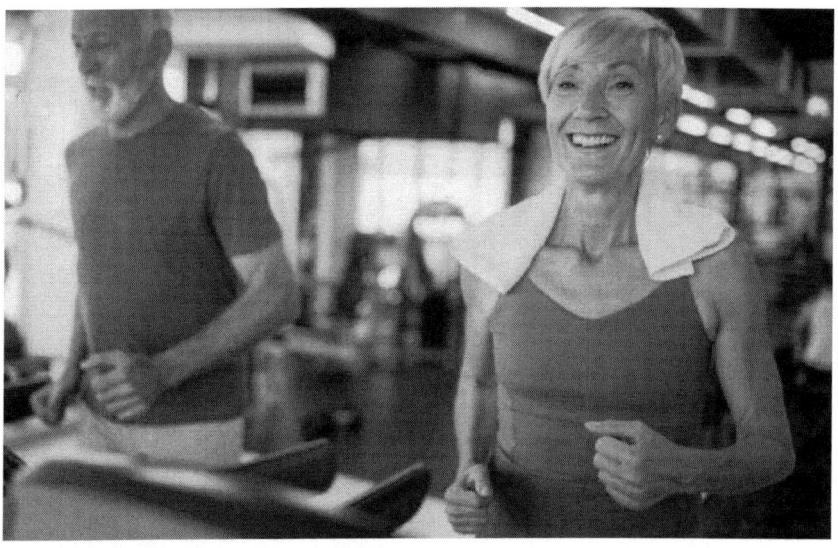

Weeks Seven to Twelve - Perseverance and Purpose

Twelve weeks is only eighty-four days. Ha! It's easy to say that now, at this stage, because you persevered.

TIP: During your six week follow-up appointment with the surgeon, share what you would like to be doing in the near future. What is something you haven't been able to do? For me, it was snowshoe hiking. I had my THR (total hip replacement) in early winter, in Alaska where I live. With all the cold weather, short days and darkness, it's important for one's sanity to get outside and enjoy the world around. Otherwise you get what we call 'cabin fever.'

I shared this with my doctor and she confirmed that I would be ready for this challenge by week twelve.

THAT kept me going. Find that thing that will help you persevere through the final stages of recovery...with a hopeful attitude.

Purpose: /ˈpərpəs/ noun

the reason for which something is done or created or for which something exists.
   "the purpose of THR is to live fully again, doing the things that make you happy"

Similar: motive, motivation, objective, goal, benefit, outcome, function
   ~ **Oxford Languages**

6

CONCLUSION

Celebrate Success!

If you have read this and are contemplating total hip replacement surgery, I hope this gave you enough insight to make your own conclusion.

Yes, it's scary.
　Yes, it's a commitment.
　Yes, you'll have to sacrifice some time.
　Yes, you'll feel frustrated at times.
　Yes, you'll feel renewed hope at other times.
　Yes, it's absolutely worth it!

I wish you all the luck in your journey.

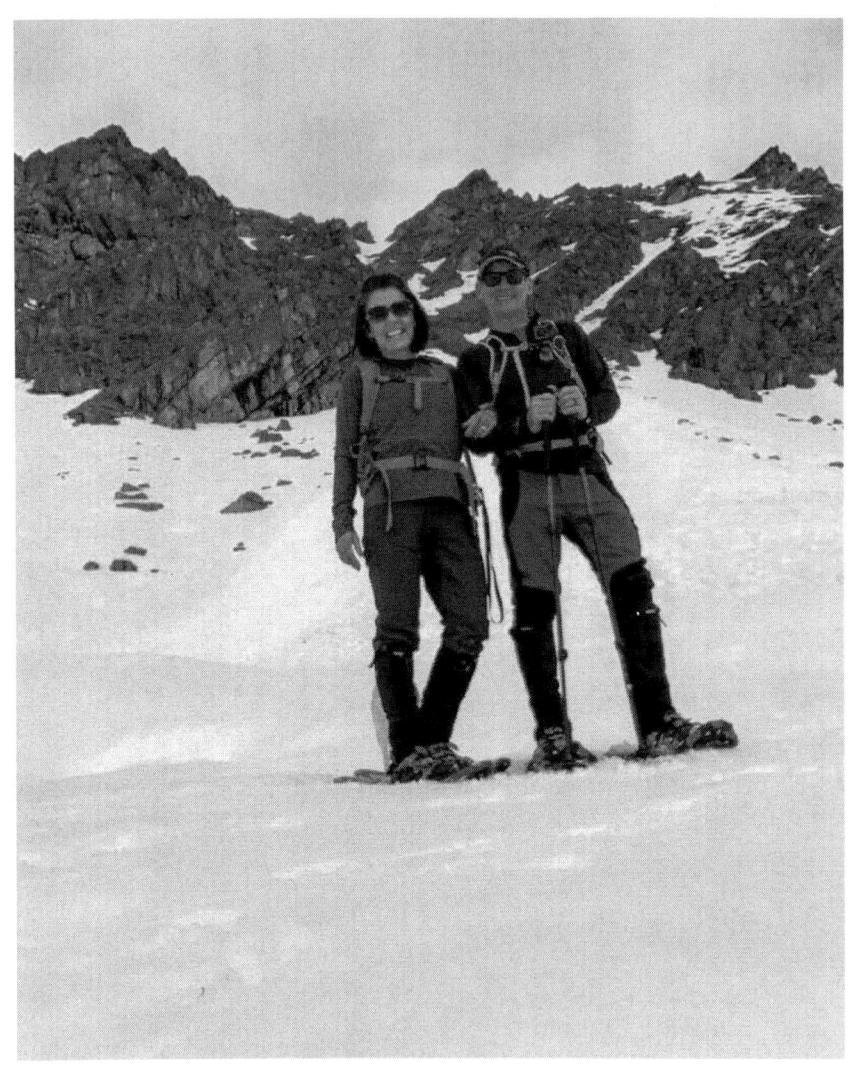

7

RESOURCES

Hip Arthritis. (2022, January 7). Johns Hopkins Medicine. https://www.hopkinsmedicine.org/health/conditions-and-diseases/hip-arthritis

Nottoli, C. (2019, December 16). The Hip is the Largest, Strongest Joint in the Human Body. Functional Pain Relief. https://www.functionalpainrelief.com/patient-education/2018/7/9/the-hip-is-the-largest-strongest-joint-in-the-human-body

Gastritis - Symptoms and causes. (2022, March 15). Mayo Clinic. https://www.mayoclinic.org/diseases-conditions/gastritis/symptoms-causes/syc-20355807

Jenkinson, C. (2016, May 10). Definition, Measures, Applications, & Facts. Encyclopedia Britannica. https://www.britannica.com/topic/quality-of-life

Foran, J.H.R, MD, FAAOS. (2022, June). Total Hip Replacement. https://orthoinfo.aaos.org/. Retrieved December 26, 2022, from https://orthoinfo.aaos.org/en/treatment/total-hip-replacement/

DeSantis, C. (2022, January 21). Questions To Ask Before Hip Replacement Surgery. Advanced Orthopedics New England. https://www.ctortho.com/2022/01/20/questions-to-ask-before-hip-replacement-surgery/

Northwestern Medicine. (n.d.). Prosthetic Joint Infections Causes and Diagnoses. https://www.nm.org/conditions-and-care-areas/infectious-disease/prosthetic-joint-infections/causes-and-diagnoses

Benefits of owning a life insurance policy to cover your final expenses. (n.d.). State Farm. https://www.statefarm.com/simple-insights/life-insurance/guaranteed-life-insurance

Total Hip Replacement (Direct Anterior Approach). (2022, October 30). Yale Medicine. https://www.yalemedicine.org/conditions/total-hip-replacement-anterior-approach

Anterior vs. Posterior Hip Replacement Surgeries. (n.d.). Arthritis-health. https://www.arthritis-health.com/surgery/hip-surgery/anterior-vs-posterior-hip-replacement-surgeries

Printed in Dunstable, United Kingdom